THE NATURAL REMEDY FOR TOOTH DECAY

HOW TO REMEDY TOOTH DECAY NATURALLY IN THE COMFORT OF YOUR OWN HOME

D1437471

KATE EVANS SCOTT

KATE EVANS SCOTT

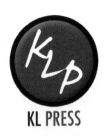

KL PRESS

DISCLAIMER

KATE EVANS SCOTT

This book is dedicated to everyone who seeks to live their healthiest life.

KATE EVANS SCOTT

ACKNOWLEDGMENTS

Thank You to my friends and family for your encouragement.
Your support has been the cornerstone of this creative process.

A special thanks also goes out to you the reader ~ I am
grateful to be sharing this journey to health and happiness
together with you.

CONTENTS

CONTENTS

KATE EVANS SCOTT

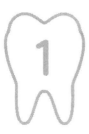

NATURAL TOOTH CARE: PREVENT AND REVERSE CAVITIES

The only way to fix a cavity is to scrape it out and fill it, right? Wrong. That's what your dentist tells you, and what he or she may actually believe. But the reality is that we can heal and strengthen our teeth from the inside out using proper nutrition and alternative care practices.

Despite the fact that modern culture has separated dental from medical practices to the point that even insurance coverage is separate, our teeth are still just as much a part of our bodies as our blood, bones and organs!

Your teeth are positioned at the end of a very long and elaborate system of nerves, cells, and tissues that work to keep them healthy and strong. In fact, some of the first signs of disease are found in the teeth and gums... I'm sure you've heard the news that gum health is linked to cardiovascular disease!

It makes absolutely no sense to separate dental health from the rest of your body's wellbeing.

We, as a culture, are doing it wrong and it shows. According to research published by the National Institute of Dental and Craniofacial Research, the numbers show an alarming upward trend in tooth decay since the 1990's [1] :

> 42% of children aged 2 – 11 have dental caries in their primary teeth, and 21% have decay in permanent teeth
> 42% of adults aged 35 – 44 have decayed, missing, or filled teeth

MOST SHOCKING: There is only a 1% drop in decayed, missing, or filled teeth when the demographic drops below the poverty line. [2]

The U.S. spends over $20 billion per year on dental care.

With the level of technology available to us getting increasingly more advanced, and access to dental care rising along with availability of knowledge regarding tooth health, why isn't the rate of cavitation dropping? Interestingly enough, that answer could be right in front of us: diet. It can't possibly be coincidence that the rise in cavities runs parallel to the rise in processed food consumption in our grab-no-go dining culture.

If you are eating what you consider a healthy diet, but you have a new cavity each time you go to the dentist, it's probably not because you have poor dental hygiene. **Ninety percent of American adults have cavities in almost half of their teeth.** The percentage of kids' teeth with cavities is rising at an alarming rate—which makes no sense if it's just a matter of brushing and flossing.

Dr. William Bowen, D.D.S., Ph.D., Professor of Dentistry at the University of Rochester, is an internationally recognized authority on tooth decay. In an article released in 2000, he shows his alarm regarding the rise in tooth decay[3] : *"Ninety-five percent of adults have cavities. Some people have the idea that the problem has been solved, but that's ridiculous. There is no other disease I know of where it's considered success when 50 percent or more of the population still has the disease."*

Dental caries in children were steadily declining through the 1970's and 80's, but research now shows that cavities have risen drastically in recent years—jumping from an average of two cavities in the mouths of ten year olds to three!

That's an increase of 33%! Dental hygiene alone cannot possibly account for all of these cavities. When your properly brushed tooth shows dental caries, more likely than not it is because your teeth aren't getting the food they need to remineralize and stay strong.

WHAT EXACTLY ARE CAVITIES, AND HOW DO WE GET THEM?

A cavity is a hole in the tooth enamel. "Dental caries" is another name for cavities. Once the enamel has a hole in it, bacteria get in there and rot out the tooth pulp, eventually killing the tooth. Okay, that's pretty simple, but the bigger question is this: *what causes cavities?* Herein lies the problem.

The modern practice of dentistry upholds a scientific theory that cavities are primarily caused by bacteria on the teeth. The reality is that this theory was *adopted by vote* decades ago and *has not been irrevocably proven*. Meanwhile, other theories with a great deal of evidence to back them have been dismissed—this includes the concept that **tooth decay is caused primarily by poor diet**, not by acid or bacteria left on the teeth.

Maverick dentist, Dr. Weston Price, developed his nutrition theory after travelling the globe studying cultures that either had low rates of dental caries or high. He focused a lot of his research on primitive people, disconnected from the luxury of convenience foods, as these people seemed to have the best teeth and overall health. Paying close attention to their diet and dental hygiene, he found something striking: People who ate a traditional diet including whole foods high in fat-soluble vitamins and minerals with little or no processed grains and sugars **had almost no cavities.**

Wait, there's more: People eating this type of diet had healthy, strong teeth regardless of dental hygiene! Cultures that were introduced to modern convenience foods including jams and jellies, pastries, white bread, and abundant sugary fruits had far worse teeth even if their dental hygiene was good! Dr. Price took his hypothesis that poor nutrition caused cavities straight to the lab, testing foods for their nutritional content and conducting a series of studies to prove his theory.

In one case, Price studied a group of poor children who subsisted mainly on a diet that "...usually consisted of highly sweetened strong coffee and white bread, vegetable fat, pancakes made of white flour and eaten with syrup, and doughnuts fried in vegetable fat." This diet was lacking the fat-soluble vitamins and minerals necessary for building strong teeth... and these children had the decayed teeth to prove it!

Dr. Price set out to nourish the children's bodies so that their teeth would remineralize, heal the cavities, and prevent future dental caries. This would provide a solid foundation for his hypothesis. For the purposes of the study, these malnourished children were fed a nutrient rich diet for one meal, six days per week, for five months.

In this excerpt from his revolutionary book, *Nutrition and Physical Degeneration: A Comparison of Primitive and Modern Diets and Their Effects*, Dr. Price details the cavity-reversing menu:

*The nutrition provided to these children in this one meal included the following foods. About four ounces of **tomato juice or orange juice** and a teaspoonful of a mixture of equal parts of a very high vitamin **natural cod liver oil** and an especially **high vitamin butter** was given at the beginning of the meal. They then received a bowl containing approximately a pint of a very **rich vegetable and meat stew, made largely from bone marrow** and fine cuts of tender meat: the meat was usually broiled separately to retain its juice and then chopped very fine and added to the bone marrow meat soup which always contained finely chopped vegetables and plenty of very yellow carrots; for the next course they had cooked fruit, with very little sweetening, and **rolls made from freshly ground whole wheat**, which were spread with the **high-vitamin butter**. The wheat for the rolls was ground fresh every day in a motor driven coffee mill. Each child was also given **two glasses of fresh whole milk**. The menu was varied from day to day by substituting for the meat stew, **fish chowder or organs of animals**.*

Miraculously, the children's dental caries halted-- and x-rays showed the teeth healing and strengthening! Through this and other studies, Dr. Price maintained his hypothesis that not only is tooth decay caused by malnutrition, but that it can be prevented and reversed through proper nutrition.

The bottom line is: Plugging cavities doesn't heal teeth. Nourishing foods heal teeth.

In fact, fillings block the proper flow of nutrients to the teeth. Sure, a filling will remove and stop the decay, but it ultimately kills the tooth. The evidence to that affect is apparent when you go to the dentist and find that you need to have an old filling replaced... or worse, many root canals are performed on teeth that have previously been filled! While they can be a helpful tool in severe cases of decay, fillings are a temporary fix for a deeper-seeded problem.

To set the record straight, I am not suggesting that proper nutrition will grow new tooth material to fill in holes caused by dental caries.

Just like with your bones, once the bit of tooth is lost, it's gone. However, when your body is filled with the proper fat-soluble nutrients, your teeth will harden and turn glassy around the cavities, protecting the pulp inside from bacteria and infection. This will essentially seal your tooth naturally, and your teeth will be strong enough to resist future caries.

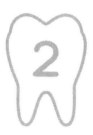

THE RIGHT DIET FOR TOOTH HEALTH

I can tell you that the proper diet can heal your teeth all I want, but what's the proper diet? We are inundated with every kind of diet plan from low fat and vegan, to high-protein and low-carb. We have diet books with thin celebrities on the front, and ones with the guys sporting six-pack abs. The term "healthy diet" can be really confusing.

For the purposes of this book, we are going to limit the conversation to a diet that promotes healthy teeth. Having said that, the reason tooth health improves on this plan is because your entire body is satiated with nourishing vitamins and minerals from:

Fresh and cooked vegetables
Pasture-raised meat (including organ meat), poultry and eggs
Raw and fermented pastured-raised dairy
Bone broth
Seafood and cod liver oil

Healthy body, healthy teeth. This is a holistic approach that has been used in eastern and traditional medical practice for thousands of years, but has been lost on modern civilization. How does it work? The mechanism for healing teeth with nutrition is pretty straightforward.

Your teeth are composed of four main substances: Enamel, dentin, pulp, and cementum.

Enamel: This is the hard layer on the outside of the crown portion of the tooth. It's the hardest substance in the body, which is necessary to handle all of the chewing we do every day. *It is believed in modern dentistry that tooth enamel isn't able to resist acid, which eats holes through it if left unchecked.*

Dentin: This layer is just below the enamel and is similar to bone. Its softer composition allows it to distribute the pressure of each bite.

Pulp: This is the innermost layer of the tooth. It's the soft substance which houses the nerves and provides nutrients to the rest of the tooth. When a tooth is decayed, the pulp has begun to rot away.

Cementum: This is located around the root of the tooth and attaches the tooth to the bone.

When the body becomes satiated with the proper level of fat-soluble vitamins and minerals, it will send the necessary nutrients to the pulp of the teeth, which will then supply the enamel, dentin, and cementum with what they need to strengthen and heal. This process is called remineralization. However, if the body has been depleted of these vital nutrients, or is unable to absorb them, the teeth are the last in line for distribution.

In Dr. Price's observations, the cultures who showed the worst cases of cavitation had a diet that was not only full of sugars and grain, but was devoid of fat-soluble **Vitamins A and D and essential enamel-building minerals.**

Meats that are fed on green grasses, as well as free-range chicken and duck eggs, raw milk, soups made from boiling marrow bones, and fresh seafood, fill the body with healthy doses of these fat-soluble vitamins and minerals (such as phosphorus) that stimulate the glands and send vital nutrients to the teeth.

Now, the food we eat is dictated by the Big Food Industry's bottom line and our highly refined taste buds. In a culture that is moving further away from natural, whole foods and closer to a diet largely composed of chemicals and processed food-products, we are becoming incredibly unhealthy in our bodies, minds, and our mouths.

ORGAN MEATS:

You or your parents may have grown up eating liver and onions. Now, most of us snub our noses at consuming the internal organs of animals. But the fact is that the livers, hearts, brains, intestinal walls, blood, and pancreas of humanely raised free-range animals are full of vital nutrients for not only tooth health, but whole body wellness.

Organic liver provides over 400 % of the USDA recommended daily allowance of fat-soluble Vitamin A, and 30 % of Vitamin D, along with a healthy dose of phosphorus and other minerals. These nutrients are a vital component in the process of tooth remineralization.[4]

Primitive cultures, including Native Americans, understood the value of consuming the entire animal. They would roast and eat every organ, and crack the bones for the nutrient-rich marrow. In fact, children were often fed on a broth made from marrow as a compliment to or substitute for their mother's milk.

If you're feeling uncomfortable with cooking liver, try this simple trick: Make a meatloaf with grass-fed ground beef, chopped onion, free-range egg, and a few ounces of finely chopped liver. Cook as you normally would, or make it into patties and cook like you would a burger or meatballs.

The blended textures of the meat mixture will mask the smoother texture of the liver, and the flavors will blend nicely. As you get more used to the strong, earthy liver flavor, you can increase the amount of organ meat in your mixture.

BONE BROTH:

Bone broth isn't as gory as it may sound. It is simply a broth made from slow-cooking the bones from free-range, grass-fed animals; or whole fish or crustacean carcasses.

Bone broths contain a high quantity of vital minerals including calcium, phosphorous, magnesium, sulfur, fluoride, sodium and potassium. These minerals, especially phosphorous, are essential for rebuilding the mineral structure of the teeth.

In order to attack cavities from the inside out, I suggest eating or drinking 2 – 3 cups of bone broth per day. You can use it to make a hearty stew, or simply drink it from a mug. Either way, the gelatin, fat-soluble vitamins and minerals are getting into your body to help the rebuilding process.

To make bone broth, simply place the bones or entire carcass of a free-range fowl, a bovine marrowbone, or fish carcass into the slow cooker with a splash of vinegar. Fill to the top with fresh water and sea salt (optional). Set the slow cooker to low, replace the lid, and let simmer for 24 – 48 hours.

Real bone broth will become gelatinous when refrigerated, and makes very good thick soups and gravies as well as bases for traditional soups like chicken and vegetable or beef-mushroom. Remember to steer clear of noodles or other grains in your soups, but adding diced vegetables is absolutely okay!

COD LIVER OIL:

Fermented cod-liver oil is like a liquid dentist—only much less frightening. (Seriously, who doesn't cringe a bit when the dentist gets out that scraper?) Full of highly concentrated fat-soluble vitamins A & D, just ½ teaspoon 2 – 3 times a day can immediately alleviate tooth pain. Why? Because you're sending a rush of nutrients to your teeth that are an integral part of structural repair.

STOP: Don't go running to your health food store or hop on Amazon to buy a bottle of cod liver oil just yet. It's crucial to remember that **not all cod liver oil is created equal.** *Fermented* cod liver oil is not exposed to the high heats often used when processing commercial oils. Heat processing completely obliterates naturally occurring vitamin D, which has to then be added back in synthetic form—which is essentially not absorbable by the human body.

One of the most reliable sources of fermented cod liver oil is Green Pasture's Blue Ice Fermented Cod Liver Oil found online at the **codliveroilshop.com**. The web site recommends that you take the cod liver oil with high vitamin butter oil... which brings us to the next food on your tooth-health diet plan.

GRASS-FED BUTTER OR GHEE:

Remember when butter was the bad guy? Well, delicious, creamy, fatty butter isn't totally off the hook. Those hunks of pale butter found in most grocers' refrigerators are NOT going to help heal your teeth.

Factory-farmed dairy can't even nourish a calf, let alone a human being.

Commercial butter is made from milk that is pumped from grain-fed, confined cows that are generally treated with hormones and antibiotics. It has none of what Dr. Price called Activator X—a property found only in dairy from cows that were grazed on the rapidly growing grasses in the spring and early summer. This grass-fed butter is a deep yellow color and is full of fat-soluble vitamins A, K, and E. It's got a great balance of Omega-6 to Omega-3 fatty acids[5], and it has that mysterious "Activator X."

According to Dr. Price's research, "Many children have tooth decay even while using whole milk, in part because the milk is too low in vitamin content, due to the inadequacy of the food given the cows." He also explains that rapidly-growing grass-fed "...butter is usually several times as high in fat-soluble activators including vitamins A and D as butter produced from stall fed cattle or cattle on poorer pasturage." [6]

He found that people who ate a diet including plenty of grass-fed butter were very healthy with almost no cavities, and that the rate of dental caries decreases during the spring and summer when butter is made from the milk of cows grazing on young green grasses. This is because the deep yellow pastured dairy contains a component that activates the body's ability to absorb minerals—"Activator X."

Better mineral absorption means greater tooth mineralization. If you have lactose intolerance, you can use ghee instead of butter. Ghee is simply butter that has been clarified by heating it up and skimming off the water and milk solids. It's free of lactose and casein, and it really adds delicious flavor to your foods. PLUS, it increases essential vitamin absorption. Remember to only use ghee that is organic and grass-fed, which can be found at most health food stores.

Or you can make your own ghee from pastured butter: Place a pound of organic, pastured butter (such as Kerrigold) into a Dutch oven or other oven-safe dish. Turn oven to 250°F and bake for about an hour. At this point, check on the ghee—it should be very bubbly and browning on the bottom. Continue baking for about another 30 minutes until slightly toasted on the bottom, but not burned.

Remove from the oven and let the ghee cool slightly so it's easier to handle. Line a fine mesh sieve with a couple layers of cheesecloth or a clean muslin cloth and set it over a large bowl. Gently pour the ghee through the cheesecloth, collecting the solids in the cloth. Pour the clear liquid ghee into a clean Mason jar and store in a cool, dry place.

If you aren't interested in either of these options, you can always add the high vitamin butter oil (Green Pasture's) to your daily dose of cod liver oil.

FERMENTED FOODS:

Eating raw vegetables isn't necessarily nutritionally superior. Just because you can chow down on raw broccoli doesn't mean you're healthier, it just means you can really chew.

It might be a good idea to replace that raw broccoli slaw, which is a bit difficult to digest, with sauerkraut. Fermented foods such as raw milk kefir and yogurt, sauerkraut, kimchi, pickles, and kombucha contain enzymes that have already started the process of breaking food down before it even hits your mouth. This is important because fermentation eases the absorption of nutrients into the body.[7]

The active cultures in real, traditionally-fermented foods are considered probiotics, promoting the growth of healthy bacteria in the gut and thus increasing the absorption of vital nutrients such as the B vitamins, which we already know are essential for tooth remineralization. [9]

The most important thing to remember when picking pickles are the words "traditionally fermented." If a container of pickles or olives or kraut doesn't say that it contains **active cultures**, then it's probably commercially processed and will have no positive effects on your gut flora.

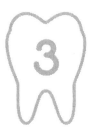

REMOVING GRAINS AND SUGAR

Do you know how many parents say that their children only eat white things? We're talking about pasta, bread, pastries, potatoes, sugar... all nutritionally void foods that do more to damage your health than nourish your body. But I'm telling you right now that it is easier than you think to cut them out of your life once you realize the damage they are causing.

Your dentist is kind of right. Staying away from sugary snacks and grain products is good advice, but perhaps not for the reasons your dentist leads you to think.

THE WHOLE GRAIN FALLACY:

Back in the early 1900's, the American Dental Association adopted a theory that acids sitting on your teeth were the root cause of cavities. While this theory was grounded in scientific research, it was not fully proven nor should it have trumped the other theories being developed at the time. However, the Acid Theory was taken for truth and has since dominated dental practices in the developed world.

Right around the same time that Dr. Price was researching the relationship between nutrition and decay in the early 1900's, Drs. Edward and May Mellanby, a husband and wife team, were studying the effects of whole grains on dental caries and the development of rickets.

We are lead to believe that whole grains are healthy. Those people who follow a Paleo diet remove all grains for a number of reasons, the primary health benefit being a reduction in low-grade inflammation.

A secondary benefit, which is no less important, is that removing grains from the diet allows for better absorption of fat-soluble vitamins crucial for protecting and healing teeth.

During the course of their extensive research on the cause and cure for rickets, the Mellanby's discovered that unsoaked whole grains are high in phytic acid, which effectively **inhibits the absorption of essential vitamins and minerals** including vitamin D, calcium, and phosphorus.[8] Remember that these are the building blocks of healthy tooth remineralization. Rickets is also caused by a lack of these vitamins and minerals and often results in skeletal deformation, bone fractures, muscle weakness, and **dental problems**.

During the vast famine in the early 20th century, rickets was an epidemic among impoverished children. Now, even our wealthy children are nutritionally starved. The only difference is that this malnutrition has manifested in their mouths, instead of the full range of symptoms often accompanying rickets.

By removing grains from the diet, you increase absorption of fat-soluble vitamins and minerals which leads to stronger, healthier teeth that are able to resist acids and the resulting bacteria indefinitely.'

THE BITTER TRUTH ABOUT SUGAR

We all know that sugar is bad for us. It makes us fat, sick, pale, depressed, moody, and it rots our teeth. So why are we consuming it in such ridiculous quantities? In 2013, **Americans consumed over ten million metric tons of sugar**. To break it down for you, that's **between 80 – 100 pounds of sugar per person,** per year. Can you imagine eating nearly half of a one-pound bag of sugar every few days?

Well, if you're anything like the average American surviving on the modern diet, you are doing just that. No, you're not sitting under the table with a bag of sugar and a big spoon. The sugar is hidden in all of the processed convenience foods that have replaced the slow-cooked real meals that were the diet mainstay of generations that came before us.

Processed white sugar has been stripped of any nutrients it may have once contained, then it's concentrated until it's very sweet. While half of your average sugar intake is from the obvious items like soda, cookies, candy, and ice cream, the rest is **deeply hidden in foods you may never suspect—yes, even the "organic" and "natural" ones**. Check the labels closely, you'll find sugar added to unlikely food items, such as: pasta sauce, fish sticks, catsup, soy, almond milks, soups, breads, cereals, and many more. Our modern processed diet is full of it -- there are added processed sugars in ¾ of the 600,000 grocery items in the average super market! [10]

But you read the label, and it doesn't say "sugar!" Right. That's how sneaky sugar hides right before your very eyes. Sugar has as many as **fifty-six aliases**. Some of these alternative names for sugar include:

Brown rice syrup
High fructose corn syrup
Fructose
Lactose
Maltodextrin
Malt syrup
Dextrose

Demarara sugar
Molasses
Raw sugar
Sorbitol
Treacle

Just because the label doesn't say "sugar," doesn't mean it's sugar-free. That's the tricky part. Even *grape or apple juice concentrate* has the same effect on your body as straight-up sugar.... So put back those all-natural gummy fruit snacks and go for a pint of strawberries instead!

Why is sugar so bad? Well, traditional dentistry will defer to the *acid and bacteria theory*. Your dentist has probably told you not to suck on hard candies or drink soda because the sugar will sit on your teeth and chew a hole through your enamel, thus making way for bacteria to infect the tooth pulp and rot your tooth. Sound familiar?

This is true, and also misleading. A truly healthy and nourished tooth will be able to resist that sugar invasion indefinitely. Even the doctor responsible for developing the acid theory of cavitation, Dr. Miller himself, said that *a perfectly healthy tooth would resist cavitation indefinitely*. The problem is that the sugar doesn't just sit on your teeth. It goes into your body as well. When you combine the sugar sitting in your mouth with the fact that sugar is absorbing into your body, you create a monster.

Sugar, along with all of its pseudonyms, is ultimately processed in the liver, unlike sugar's healthier counterpart—glucose, which is turned into energy in the body. If you are consuming the average 80 – 100 pounds of processed sugar per year, you are going to very quickly overload your liver. **Once the liver is overloaded, it can't do one of its many important jobs: breaking down the fat-soluble vitamins A,D,E, and K!** If the liver isn't breaking down those vitamins, they're not getting to your teeth.

If the vitamins aren't getting to your teeth, your teeth will become malnourished and weak.

When your teeth are malnourished and weak, they will not be able to withstand the sugars sitting on them.

The result is a vicious cycle of sugar-malabsorption-cavity, sugar-malabsorption-cavity.

Driven almost exclusively by profits, the foods industry knows what it's doing by filling products full of sugar—**they are creating addictions**. The more sugar you eat, the more you want, and ultimately the more of their product you're going to buy. It's a simple supply-and-demand cycle that we have allowed to fundamentally change the way we eat and feed our families.

We have become accustomed to a higher level of sweetness to our foods than nature intended. Our choices are being driven by our taste buds, which is a very bad thing. An overloaded liver not only contributes to tooth decay, but it also turns sugar straight into fat instead of your body converting it into accessible energy.

So, the simple equation is this: Sugar causes bacteria to produce enamel-eating acid PLUS sugar prevents the absorption of remineralizing nutrients = fragile, malnourished teeth that can't resist decay.

Now, when your dentist tells you to stay away from sugar, you'll know the entire reason why—not just one end of the cycle. Think about it... if sugar is only responsible for bacteria eating holes in teeth, you should be able to brush it off and be fine... but the skyrocketing increase in the rate of dental caries in cultures that subsist on a modern, processed diet proves that it just doesn't work that way.

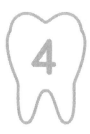

HOMEOPATHY FOR
HEALTHY TEETH

The term "homeopathy" is derived from the Greek words meaning "like" and "suffering." Homeopathic practitioners claim that homeopathy dates all the way back to 400 B.C. when Hypocrates prescribed very small doses of mandrake root to cure mania... knowing very well that large doses of mandrake root actually *causes* mania.

Sounds a bit ludicrous, right? Well, if you think so, you're not alone. Homeopathy has been scrutinized since its inception. It's been called quackery and nothing more than a placebo effect. However, thousands of people across many cultures swear by it and use it regularly to heal their bodies, minds, and teeth.

What is homeopathy? In the practice of homeopathy, very diluted amounts of a substance is given to heal precisely what a larger dose may exacerbate—as in the mandrake example. Homeopathic remedies are made by diluting a substance in alcohol or distilled water until there are actually very few or no molecules of that initial substance remaining. This diluted solution is then given, generally in tablet form that is held under the tongue, to heal a specific malady.

This thousands-year-old practice was revitalized by Samuel Hahnemann in the early 1800's.[11] He postulated his theory that "like cures like" when noticing that a medicine designed to cure a disease in an infected person often causes a healthy individual similar symptoms to that very disease. During the time that Hahnemann was developing his homeopathic ideas and formulating remedies, popular medical practice consisted of mixtures containing long lists of harmful drugs and chemicals, such as opium and viper's blood. Bloodletting and purging were common as well.

Hahnemann believed these somewhat barbaric yet popular medical practices to be harmful rather than healing—in fact, a lot of people died after receiving painful medical treatment during that time. This is likely the reason that some people started turning to Hahnemann's homeopathic methods, which focused on low doses of single "medications" or remedies as an alternative to the almost barbaric practices that often lead to a worsening of symptoms or even death. Hahnemann believed that diseases also had a non-tangible, spiritual quality that could be addressed with his homeopathic remedies.

The second principle separating homeopathic methodology from modern medical practice is the belief that the lower the dosage of a remedy, the more effective. This is why the original substance is so extremely diluted that often times it's merely the "essence" of that substance remaining in the solution.

Since Hahnemann published his book of 65 homeopathic remedies, *Materia Medica Pura*, in 1810, homeopathy has spread throughout the world as an alternative to mainstream medicine. Even though scientific research to back the efficacy of homeopathy is lacking, millions of people turn to this gentler healing method:

"According to the 2007 National Health Interview Survey, which included a comprehensive survey of the use of complementary health practices by Americans, an estimated 3.9 million adults and 910,000 children used homeopathy in the previous year. These estimates include use of over-the-counter products labeled as "homeopathic," as well as visits with a homeopathic practitioner. Out-of-pocket costs for adults were $2.9 billion for homeopathic medicines and $170 million for visits to homeopathic practitioners."[12]

Homeopathy's holistic view of the body is consistent with our plan of treating our teeth as a part of the entire being, rather than a separate entity requiring an entirely different medical practice and approach.

CALC FLUOR AND CALC PHOS FOR TOOTH REMINERALIZATION

Calc fluor and **calc phos** are the common homeopathic names for *calcium fluoride and calcium phosphorus.* These are two of the twelve basic cell salts, minerals that make up the building blocks of the body and provide a foundation for enzyme activity.

Calcium Fluoride (Calc fluor): Calcium is absolutely essential for building strong bones and teeth—but unfortunately this vital mineral is lacking in the modern diet of sugars and starches. When the body is deficient in calcium, it will actually leach minerals from the bones to supply the rest of the body. Calcium Fluoride (not to be confused with its potentially harmful cousins Fluorosilicic Acid and Sodium Fluorosilicate found in most tap water), is a naturally occurring mineral that binds with your tooth enamel, strengthening teeth against harmful bacteria. It can be an effective treatment for preventing tooth decay.

Calcium fluoride is responsible for: elasticity, flexibility, toning; strength and resilience in muscular and connective tissues, bones, tooth enamel, and blood vessel walls.[13]

Calcium Phosphorus (Calc phos): As we have already discussed, our modern diets are often starving us of vital nutrients. We are mineral deficient, and most importantly for tooth health, we lack the necessary calcium and phosphorus to remineralize our teeth and protect them from decay.

The tissue salt *calc phos* contributes to: the building of cells; is an essential component of blood, connective tissues, teeth, and bones; provides general maintenance for body function, support for recuperation, growth, and development.[14]

85% of our body's phosphorus can be found in the bones and teeth. However, those concentrations are greatly depleted when the body is deficient of phosphorus elsewhere.[15] *Calc phos* is a homeopathic low-dose of calcium and phosphorus designed to help replenish those essential minerals.

If you are maintaining the diet outlined in this book, rich in raw milk, fermented cod liver oil, bone broth and grass-fed meats with no grains or sugar, you should be able to maintain a healthy level of calcium, phosphorous, and fluoride to uphold the integrity of your teeth. However, in some occasions—especially in the case of growing children—teeth experience weakened enamel and decay despite the healthy diet described in previous chapters of this book. In those cases, adding in the recommended dosage of homeopathic *calc fluor* **and** *calc phos* **can help your body rejuvenate the teeth naturally** and without mainstream dental intervention. Once the decayed teeth have been restored, you can ease off of the homeopathic cell salts as recommended by your homeopath.

The *calc fluor* and *calc phos* homeopathic remedies come in the form of tiny white tablets that taste a little bit sweet when held under the tongue, making them perfect for small children. The gums and tongue are highly absorbent, which means these mineral salts rush straight into the blood stream and get right to work rebuilding the teeth.

Supplementing with homeopathic remedies is especially good in cases where you are noticing brown or gray spots on the teeth of very young children that are already consuming a tooth-healthy diet. *Homeopathic remedies are not intended as a replacement for the diet.* You cannot continue to feed your child with a diet full of sugar and starch, lacking vital nutrients, and then expect to heal them with homeopathic remedies. This is just one tool included in a comprehensive plan to go after particularly problematic teeth.

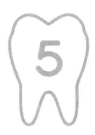

ELIMINATING TOXIC TOOTHPASTE

When you stand at the grocery store and look at the wall of toothpastes, you'll see lots of claims that this one will whiten teeth or that one will strengthen enamel. What all of that clever packaging doesn't share is the laundry list of toxic chemicals filling the tube. Even though you're brushing, rinsing, and spitting the toothpaste out, those toxins get absorbed through your gums almost the moment they make contact.

Below are a few of the toxic chemicals found in many of the commercial toothpastes. Are you surprised? If you've ever read a toothpaste label, you'd know that it states clearly: Do NOT swallow. That's because swallowing this product—which is intended to put in the mouth, remember—*could be dangerous*.

Diethanolamine (DEA) is a foaming agent found in a large number of personal care products, from shampoo to hand soap, shave cream to (yep) toothpaste. *Apparently, we like things that foam.* While those bubbles might help you feel like you're getting a better clean, the chemical DEA is hugely detrimental to your health and counteracts the intention of using toothpaste in the first place—**it's ultimately not good for tooth health**! Why? Because DEA disrupts normal kidney and liver function. As discussed in previous chapters, proper kidney function is integral to processing the minerals necessary to send nutrients to the teeth. Injure kidney function and the teeth will not properly remineralize.

Triclosan is an antibacterial agent found in many toothpaste brands. While its toxicity isn't aimed specifically at disturbing functions that relate directly to tooth health, we now understand that healthy teeth are just one part of a whole healthy body. When the rest of the immune system is attacked or suppressed, teeth will often be the first to show signs of disease.

Triclosan is a pesticide, and the Unites States Environmental Protection Agency (EPA) indicates that ingestion or exposure to this harmful chemical is threatening to human health. Furthermore, triclosan is part of a class of chemicals known as chorophenols, which are suspected of causing cancer.

Sodium laureth sulfate and sodium lauryl sulfate seem to be in almost everything you scrub, rub, or squeeze onto or into your body these days. The Environmental Working Group's (EWG) cosmetic database, Skin Deep, lists a number of high and moderate concerns with exposure to these sulfates, including: contamination with 1,4 Dioxane (a known carcinogen) during the manufacturing process; skin, eye, and lung irritation; and organ system toxicity. [16] Be careful when checking labels, because this toxin could be hiding behind a very benign-sounding name: sodium salt.

Propylene Glycol is often used as a toothpaste surfactant... and it's also used in antifreeze! Not only is propylene glycol a skin irritant, according to its Material Safety Data Sheet, it's a potential neurotoxin and could cause damage to target organs.[17]

When you start your day with a mouthful of commercial toothpaste (and even those that claim to be more "natural" at twice the price), you're setting your body up for a breakdown before you've even gotten to breakfast! But we, as a culture, have been indoctrinated to believe that these products are a necessary part of our oral hygiene routine.

While it's absolutely true that you should be keeping your teeth and mouth clean, I assure you that there are better alternatives.

BRUSHING YOUR TEETH WITH CLAY

I am not suggesting that you scoop up a clump of your children's modeling clay and start scrubbing your teeth with it. That would be disgusting, and of little use.

There are many different types of clay, and the type we are referring to when discussing tooth care is Calcium Bentonite Clay Powder—a food-grade clay that can be purchased at most health food stores or, of course, ordered online.

The health benefits of calcium bentonite clay have been understood and utilized among many cultures for centuries—only to be replaced by synthetic chemicals in the most recent of our civilized history. Since clay is essentially a mixture of minerals, metal oxides, and organic matter, it is full of health benefits for not only the teeth, but the digestive system as well. **The dental health benefits of calcium bentonite clay include:**

Absorption and elimination of toxins
Remineralization of teeth
Tooth polishing properties

You likely won't find clay toothpaste alongside the Colgate at your local grocery store. However, there is a very good clay toothpaste made by Earthworks that can be purchased at most health food stores or ordered online. It contains readily recognizable ingredients including clay and essential oils, and uses xylitol to mask the muddy flavor of the raw clay powder. Xylitol is often found in sugar-free gums and baked goods, and has recently been extolled by mainstream dentistry as a powerful tool to battle tooth decay. The best form of xylitol is extracted from birch bark—but much of the commercial grade xylitol is made from corn cob. Check the label and ask about xylitol sourcing, as elimination of corn from the diet is important for all people, and especially for those with specific corn allergies.

Making your own clay toothpaste is actually quite simple and inexpensive compared to purchasing it prepared... as is the case with most homemade foods and body care products. Here's a basic recipe to get you started:

CLAY TOOTHPASTE RECIPE

Store this natural toothpaste in a glass container with a tight-fitting lid. Avoid plastic bags or containers as the clay is very absorbent and could suck up leaching toxins from the plastics.

Ingredients:

    4 tablespoons Calcium Bentonite Clay Powder

    4 tablespoons filtered water

    2 – 4 drops mint extract, or other essential oil (optional)

    2 – 4 tablespoons birch xylitol, to taste

Directions: Gently mix all ingredients together until a smooth paste forms, adjusting water and clay as necessary to reach your preferred consistency. You can easily double or triple this recipe. Try it out with just a small amount of essential oils and xylitol, tasting as you go. You can always add more if you need it!

*If you don't want to use xylitol, or don't have access to it, use a small amount of pure liquid stevia or crushed dried stevia leaf to sweeten the paste.

To use the clay toothpaste: scoop up a small amount onto the end of your wet toothbrush. Brush your teeth with the paste using gentle circular motion, making sure to specifically address areas of concern and along the gum line.

Swish with filtered water and spit. This step is actually optional, because all of the ingredients are completely edible and actually beneficial to your digestive and immune systems.

BRUSHING WITH TOOTH SOAP

You probably think of "soap in the mouth" as a punishment for saying something naughty.... Definitely not a pleasant experience. However, using homemade tooth soap cannot only be a pleasant experience, it can help keep your teeth strong and healthy.

In his book *Good Teeth, Birth to Death* Dr. Gerald Judd, PhD recommends using bar soap to clean teeth and gums... and the idea is catching on. His rationale behind using soap over toothpaste is that most toothpastes contain glycerin, which can potentially form a coating on the teeth that takes more than twenty rinses to remove. If the tooth is covered in a tough-to-remove coating, it won't be able to absorb the necessary phosphate and calcium necessary for remineralization. According to Dr. Judd, tooth soap removes the coating from the teeth while disinfecting the gums and killing any clinging bacteria.

While you can purchase premade tooth soap, it can be quite expensive. For most people choosing to use this alternative form of tooth cleanser, it's more efficient and economic to make it at home. Here's a basic recipe that makes enough to last your whole family at least a couple of weeks:

BASIC TOOTH SOAP RECIPE

Ingredients:

4 teaspoons unscented liquid castile soap (such as Dr. Bronner's)

1/2 cup melted cold-pressed virgin coconut oil

1 to 2 tsp granulated birch xylitol or pure stevia extract to taste

25 to 30 drops antimicrobial essential oil, such as: peppermint, spearmint, cinnamon, or clove

Directions: Place 2 tablespoons of boiling water into the pitcher of your blender. Add the soap, oil, sweetener, and essential oils. Blend until light and frothy. Transfer the tooth soap to a clean pump dispenser in one of two ways: Place a funnel into the top of the dispenser and press the soap in; or, pour the soap into a large plastic bag or icing bag, cut open one small corner of the bag and essentially "pipe" the soap into the container.

To Use Tooth Soap: Squirt just a small amount of tooth soap on to your moistened brush and use as you would tooth paste.

*If you don't have access to liquid castile soap, or you prefer to use castile bar soap, just make sure that you do not use handmade soap because the glycerin generally has not been removed from the handmade soaps.

While it may take a little bit of time to get used to the taste and texture of tooth soap, you'll be inspired to stick with it once you realize that your teeth are whiter and healthier. One woman reported that her family went to regular bi-annual dental checkups and neither mom, dad, nor the two children had a single cavity in the two years since using the tooth soap, following a dental diet rich with raw milk, and supplementing with good vitamins. Prior to that, the mother reported that she would have at least one new cavity each year.

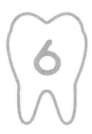

HERBAL AIDS FOR HEALTHY TEETH

The use of tiny plastic bristles attached to a plastic handle for cleaning teeth is a relatively new practice. For thousands of years, people all over the world have been cleaning their teeth with "chewing sticks." [18] The concept of the chewing sticks is not only that chewing a fibrous twig will scrape plaque off of teeth, but that the stick itself is from a plant with antimicrobial and antibacterial properties that would kill the germs before they infect the teeth.

CHEWING STICKS:

In many tribal and rural cultures all over the world, especially Africa and South America, the ends of twigs from small, fibrous bushes are shredded and used to scrub tooth surface and "floss" between teeth. While many varieties of trees and bushes have been the source of chewing sticks historically, just a few have been scientifically studied for their dental efficacy.

Two common plants still used in developing countries for general tooth care are *rhus vulgaris* and *lantana trifolia*, both of which are being studied as a possible option for providing better health care to the impoverished, as they are much cheaper and readily available than the plastic toothbrushes used in more developed industrialized parts of the world.[19]

Rhus vulgaris is commonly known by several nicknames, including Quommo and Ongafire. This small shrub produces edible berries and is found growing abundantly in Africa from Cameroon east to Ethiopia and south to Mozambique, Malawi, Zambia and Zimbabwe. [19] *Lantana trifolia* , commonly called a "shrub verbena" is a broadleaf evergreen commonly found in West Indies, Mexico, Central and South America.[20] Authors of a current research study published in *Front Pharmacol* in 2011 [21] discovered that users of chewing sticks harvested from these plants claim that:

> Cleaning posterior teeth is easier with the stick than with the modern toothbrush because the head is smaller
> The device is easier to manipulate
> The ease in cleaning individual teeth reduces instance of bleeding gums

Functionally, the sticks work really well to scrape off plaque and debris. Combining that with their innate antimicrobial properties, researchers concluded that chewing sticks are a good alternative to modern toothbrushes. With a renewed interest in alternative dental health, you can readily find dental chewing sticks for sale on the Internet and in some health food stores.

DENTAL HERBS:

The idea that diet is the primary factor in tooth decay, and subsequently tooth health, is widely accepted amongst the herbalist community. Therefore, the first thing that your herbalist will address with you when you turn to them for help with your teeth, is food. They will also complete a comprehensive set of questions about everything from your mood to your environment to better understand your individual makeup and situation. After you are thoroughly "examined," and your diet is adjusted to increase the possibility for remineralization and healing, an herbalist may direct you to several different herbs that can help give your body a tooth-building boost.

According to an article by Christopher Hobbs, LAc, AHG, an herbalist and botanist with over thirty years of experience in herbal treatments, the following herbs can help in the process of reversing pathology and strengthening teeth.[22]

ANTI-BACTERIAL & ANTI-INFLAMMATORY RESINS

The following resins contain antibacterial and anti-inflammatory properties in addition to their special characteristics listed below.

Myrrh: warming, astringent

Propolis (bee product): stimulates production of new tissue; anti-viral. Propolis is especially useful for mouth sores and ulcers.

Pine resin (pitch): can be chewed like gum when firm.

ANTI-MICROBIAL HERBS

Usnea: a common lichen, stronger than penicillin against streptococcus and staph.

Bloodroot: an eastern woodlands plant that strongly inhibits plaque and decay-causing bacteria.

Plantain: a common "weed" that can be used fresh for treatment of abscesses.

ASTRINGENTS (ANTI-MICROBIAL, TIGHTENS TISSUES)

These will help strengthen your gums and firmly root the tooth.

Krameria: contains 40% tannin (antiviral). Combine the powder with myrrh as a dentifrice for bleeding or spongy gums.

Oak galls (oak apples): contain up to 50% tannins. Use powder as a dentifrice.

Tormentil & Sage: use as a gargle for chronic gum inflammation.

IMMUNE STRENGTHENERS

A healthy immune system will ensure that your body is producing and distributing nutrients to the teeth and gums for proper healing and remineralization.

Echinacea: Gargle or rinse with the diluted tincture to activate local immunity and induce healing.

Baptisia: Antiseptic and anti-bacterial.

ESSENTIAL OILS

Most essential oil-bearing plants can stimulate blood-flow to the gums, which in turn helps drive nutrients into the teeth. The following oils are also antibacterial, so they are beneficial in removing surface bacteria:

Peppermint oil
Spearmint oil
Fennel oil
Cinnamon oil
Sage oil
Thyme oil
Oregano oil

All of these oils can be purchased easily at health food stores, can be ordered online, or obtained through your herbalist. Just make sure that your oil is of the highest quality and purity for maximum results.

KATE EVANS SCOTT

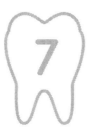

ORTHODONTICS: HOW NOT TO NEED BRACES

In the United States, braces seem almost a rite of passage... especially for the middle and upper classes. Teens and adolescents experience some shifting teeth and their dentist sends them for orthodontics. Within a few years, their teeth are straight (with or without extractions, head gear, and other appliances), their braces are removed and they go on their way—likely with some tooth decalcification.

Traditional braces straighten teeth by applying low levels of pressure, manipulated over time to move the teeth into the desired alignment. To achieve this, metal brackets are bonded directly to the tooth and then wired together and moved using elastics and springs. Sound a bit like a cyborg-smile, right? Typical braces cost between $3000 and $7000 and are not generally covered by dental insurance. [23]

PLUS, there are side-effects of braces that are almost never mentioned by your dentist, including the fact that pushing the teeth causes tooth, bone, and root damage that could lead to gum disease and root canals later in life. The potential risk of braces is always discussed in the fine print of your orthodontic contract—but does anyone really read that stuff?

Because of the high cost, the lengthy process, the appearance, or the pain of traditional braces, some parents are looking to a more holistic and natural way to straighten their teeth. This is a good thing, because simply putting braces on teeth doesn't address the root problem: *why are the teeth crooked to begin with?*

The answer is in the lifestyle of modern society. If you look at primitive cultures and our pre-industrial, pre-agricultural ancestors, there is almost no instance of crooked teeth. This is because their facial and jaw structures were perfectly wide enough to house all of the teeth—so no crowding! In his research, Dr. Weston Price noted that the diet of these primitive people was the main factor in the beautiful composition of their facial features and their healthy, straight teeth. [24]

Now, 95% of people living in countries who consume a diet mainly of processed modern foods have crooked teeth or misaligned jaws. It is important to understand that the link between diet, jaw placement, and overall health is undeniable. Dr. Price's research noted that the natives who displayed remarkably decay-free teeth also had well-formed dental arches, resulting in the wider, rounder face that is often associated with health and beauty.

When a dental arch is properly aligned, the top teeth and bottom teeth will rest flush with one another—no over bite, and no under bite. There will simply be a hairline difference with the top protruding ever so slightly so that there is not excessive pressure on the mandible. Common assumption is that crooked and misaligned teeth are genetic. We can then throw up our hands and take no responsibility. It's the easy (if not the cheap) way out.

Our modern jaws are so disfigured because of a poor diet deficient in the essential building blocks—calcium and phosphorus. This cannot be more apparent in the story of the Australian Aborigines. For thousands and thousands of years, generation after generation, these tribal Aborigines reproduced without any sign of facial irregularities such as crooked, crowded teeth or misaligned jaws... until the introduction of "white man's food" into their diet—wheat flour, grain, and sugar. **Suddenly, the children began to develop the same dental arch and facial irregularities as seen in the children of white**

civilizations. The link between diet and dental health is there and can no longer be ignored.

So, how do we prevent crooked teeth in the first place? If you've read this book through thus far, you probably know the answer: Diet.

Ideally, the **key is to begin a properly nourishing diet** prior to conception—that means you and your partner eat this way yourselves. The earlier you start nourishing the growing fetus or child properly, the better the child's chances of having a properly formed jaw and strong, straight teeth.

Once the baby is born, breastfeeding is recommended to maintain proper jaw structure and provide adequate nutrients to growing bones and developing teeth. This is an especially crucial time for the mother to nourish her own body with the same nutrient-rich diet free of sugars and grains. The fat-soluble vitamins and minerals will then be passed on to the baby through the breast milk, and mother will also reap the benefits of a healthier body and stronger teeth.

OTHER WAYS BITE AFFECTS HEALTH

A proper bite doesn't just result in *straight teeth*—it also helps you maintain strong, healthy teeth and a sound mind!

Wait, a sound mind? Yes. When your jaw is properly aligned, a whole lot of things are going on in your body:

Your airways are more open, so you breathe and sleep better. This can help with all kinds of disorders from sleep apnea to obesity, asthma, irritability, and even depression and anxiety.

Your facial structure is more appealing to potential partners (biologically speaking), so your chances of finding a mate are given a bit of a boost. Your confidence increases, and thus your relative state of happiness potentially increases. *I realize this may sound shallow and superficial, but this conclusion is drawn on anthropological evidence that potential mates are attracted to specimens of good health, which indicates healthy reproduction potential. It's survival of the fittest in action.*

Your teeth are less likely to grind or rub together, thus reducing your risk for nerve damage, cavitation, and eventually root canal.

TEETH ALREADY CROOKED?
WHAT TO DO NOW:

If your own teeth or your child's teeth are already crooked, or you are noticing an overbite or underbite, don't panic. There are steps you can take to straighten teeth and align the jaw without cementing on braces.

If your child is still very young, the first thing to do is stick very strictly to the diet outlined in this book. By starting the diet as a toddler, up to a five or six year old, you can drastically change the development of the child's bite through the food you are giving him to nourish his body. If you are addressing specific issues, you could add in the homeopathic mineral salts daily. Consult with your homeopath on types and dosages, as everyone's chemical makeup is slightly different along with other factors like age and weight.

Make sure to include plenty of raw milk products from grass-fed cows in your growing child's diet. There are different laws regulating the sale of raw milk in each individual state. However, it's fairly simple to do an internet search for "raw milk dairy" in your area and find local farms that will either allow for dairy-cow boarding or co-op milk. Ask around, check out the conditions of the farm, and get to know the farmer so that you're confident the cows are being raised properly on green pastured diet and the milk is kept sanitary. If you are unable to obtain raw milk products directly from the farm, raw cheeses are readily available at health food stores and high-end groceries.

Older children and adults should consult a Dental Orthopedic in cases of severe jaw displacement or severely crooked teeth. Unlike orthodontists, who aim to simply straighten teeth in any way possible, dental orthopedics look to align the jaw and cranium to their natural position, thus allowing for the teeth to straighten naturally without the use of braces.

In dental orthopedics, the entire cranial structure is taken into consideration rather than separating the teeth and jaw from the rest of the body.

Furthermore, dental orthopedic doctors understand the link between the cranial structure, jaw, and all of the body's intricate systems that affect every aspect of our health and well-being. As you already know, we are holistic organisms and should be considered as a whole.

According to Dr. Gerald H. Smith, "All mechanical tensions placed on the teeth will be reflected into the cranial system and if used by design can serve to correct cranial lesions and improve the patient's quality of life." [25] What he is saying is incredibly profound. Minor manipulations in wires or other appliances can apply pressure in places that will then alter other bodily systems—essentially affecting everything from physiology to psychology. Your orthopedic dentist will keep all of this in mind as he fulfills your treatment plan.

Do you think that traditional orthodontists are thinking about what other system (Nervous? Cardiovascular? Digestive?) they will affect when they tweak that wire or move that rubber band? The odds are very unlikely... not because they don't CARE, but because that's not how they were trained.

A very good orthopedic practitioner will be able to look at your entire body as a whole, incorporating bodywork like chiropractic and massage into your treatment plan. However, finding someone who looks outside the scope of his or her own expertise can be difficult. It may **ultimately be up to you** to find and explore additional treatments to address the root causes of and treatments for your jaw misalignment.

NATURAL TOOTH CARE:
YOU HAVE THE POWER

The most important thing to take from reading this book is that you are not a passive participant in your dental health. You don't simply need to sit in the dentist's chair like a victim, waiting to be lectured about oral hygiene and then drilled and filled.

Stop blaming genetics. Stop just shrugging your shoulders and shelling out for dental work you don't need. Stop thinking that fillings and braces are just a normal part of growing older.

You got yourself into this mess, you need to get yourself out.

YOU HAVE THE POWER to heal and straighten your teeth from within, and the best weapon in your arsenal is food. I understand this is a lot of information to process, and it probably requires a complete shift in your embedded beliefs about dental health. It's okay. Here are the basic guidelines outlined here for quick reference:

Eat a nutrient-rich diet including pasture-raised meat (including organ meat), poultry and eggs, raw and fermented pastured-raised dairy, bone broth, seafood and cod liver oil.

Remove sugar and grains from your diet. This is not optional.

Supplement with homeopathic cell salts and herbs when needed.

Eliminate toxic toothpaste. Instead, try using chewing sticks, tooth soap, or clay toothpaste.

Address jaw misalignment with an orthopedic dentist.

By following these basic steps, you will be able to heal your teeth from the inside out, potentially saving you thousands of dollars in dental and medical costs over the course of your lifetime. Before you know it, you'll see positive changes in both your mouth and your body.

Even if you're still skeptical, there's no risk to trying. Making these small changes is much cheaper than shelling out for dental work, it's less painful, and there are no side effects. Your teeth will become whiter, harder, and shinier. Tooth pain will disappear, and the diet will also have a positive effect on the rest of your body. You may find yourself smiling more, and feeling better.

The advice in this book is not intended to replace professional medical attention. Always consult your physician when beginning a new medical practice, especially if the goal is to target a specific medical condition. Do not discontinue taking prescribed medication without consulting your physician.

RESOURCES

1) http://www.nidcr.nih.gov/DataStatistics/
FindDataByTopic/DentalCaries/
DentalCariesChildren2to11

2) http://drc.cdc.gov/report/1_2.htm

3) http://www.urmc.rochester.edu/news/story/index.
cfm?id=-344

4) http://metabolichealing.com/organ-meats-
the-departure-from-nutrient-dense-foods-impacts-
implications/

5) http://nutritiondata.self.com/facts/
custom/2244512/2

6) http://journeytoforever.org/farm_library/price/
price16.html

7) http://www.chicagotribune.com/health/sns-
201311190000--tms--premhnstr--k-e20131120-
20131120,0,6779484.story

8) http://www.ncbi.nlm.nih.gov/pmc/articles/
PMC2520490/

9) http://articles.mercola.com/sites/articles/
archive/2004/01/03/fermented-foods-part-two.aspx

10) http://ed.ted.com/lessons/sugar-hiding-in-plain-
sight-robert-lustig

11) http://en.wikipedia.org/wiki/Homeopathy

12) http://nccam.nih.gov/health/homeopathy

13) http://tissue-salts.com/calc_fluor.html

14) http://tissue-salts.com/calc_phos.html

15) http://umm.edu/health/medical/altmed/supplement/phosphorus

16) http://www.ewg.org/skindeep/ingredient/706089/SODIUM_LAURETH_SULFATE/

17) http://www.sciencelab.com/msds.php?msdsId=9927239

18) http://www.scribd.com/doc/20941734/Miswak-Chewing-Stick-a-Cultural-and-Scientific-Heritage

19) http://www.ncbi.nlm.nih.gov/pmc/articles/PMC3108601/

20) http://www.africa.upenn.edu/faminefood/noncategorized/noncat_Rhus_vulgaris.htm

21) http://www.missouribotanicalgarden.org/PlantFinder/PlantFinderDetails.aspx?kempercode=a524

22) http://www.healthy.net/scr/Article.aspx?Id=868

23) http://health.howstuffworks.com/wellness/oral-care/kids/straighten-kids-teeth-without-braces.htm

24) http://journeytoforever.org/farm_library/price/pricetoc.html

25) http://www.icnr.com/articles/craniodontics.html

ABOUT THE AUTHOR

KATE EVANS SCOTT is the author of
the Amazon Bestselling cookbooks
The Paleo Kid, Paleo Kid Snacks, The
Paleo Kid Lunchbox and Infused: 26
Spa-Inspired Natural Vitamin Waters.

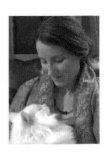

After her son was diagnosed with several
food intolerances and after having
struggled with her own Autoimmune Disease, Kate made
the commitment to remove all grains and processed
foods from her family's diet. Her passion and love for
good food blossomed after training with a retreat chef
in Belgium in her early 20's. Since then, she has wanted
to bring her love of food and health into the kitchens
of other families struggling with health and dietary
challenges.

Kate creates delicious dishes that are suitable for those
suffering from digestive and autoimmune diseases - meals
that nourish the body while healing the gut. Kate and
her husband Mark live in Oregon with their two spirited
children.

MORE BY KATE EVANS SCOTT

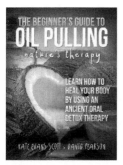

Available Now on Amazon

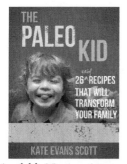

Available Now on Amazon

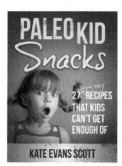

Available Now on Amazon

MORE BY KATE EVANS SCOTT

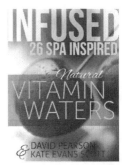

Available Now on Amazon

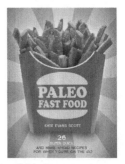

Available Now on Amazon

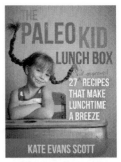

Available Now on Amazon

VISIT:

www.KidsLovePress.com

FOR MORE GREAT TITLES ON

HEALTHY LIVING!!

KATE EVANS SCOTT

29699821R00055

Made in the USA
San Bernardino, CA
26 January 2016